DR. BARBARA 7 DAYS MUCUS CLEANSE

The Simple 7- Day Plan For Mucus Cleanse And Full- Body Detox To Boost Immunity And Reset Your Body And Mind To Complete Wellness

Felicia Felix

Table of Contents

COPYRIGHT © 2023

CHAPTER ONE

Introduction to Dr. Barbara's Holistic Approach to Mucus Cleanse

Dr. Barbara's holistic approach to mucus cleanse integrates various natural healing modalities to address imbalances in the body that lea

d to excessive mucus production. This approach recognizes the interconnectedness of body systems and aims to restore balance by addressing root causes rather than just alleviating symptoms. In this comprehensive guide, we'll delve into the principles behind Dr. Barbara's approach, explore the various components involved, and discuss the benefits of adopting such a holistic perspective towards mucus cleanse.

Understanding Mucus and its Role in the Body

Before delving into Dr. Barbara's holistic approach, it's crucial to understand the role of mucus in the body. Mucus serves several essential functions, including lubricating and protecting various surfaces, such as the respiratory, digestive, and reproductive tracts. It acts as a barrier against pathogens, allergens, and irritants, helping to prevent infections and maintain overall health.

However, excessive mucus production can lead to discomfort and various health issues, including congestion, coughing, sinusitis, and digestive problems. Factors such as poor diet, dehydration, environmental toxins, and stress can contribute to increased mucus production and imbalances in the body.

The Holistic Perspective on Health and Healing

Dr. Barbara's holistic approach is rooted in the understanding that the body is a complex interconnected system, and achieving optimal health requires addressing physical, mental, emotional, and spiritual aspects. Rather than focusing solely on treating symptoms, holistic healing aims to identify and address the underlying imbalances that contribute to illness and dysfunction.

Central to the holistic perspective is the concept of the body's innate ability to heal itself when provided with the right support and conditions. This approach emphasizes the importance of lifestyle factors such as nutrition, hydration, exercise, stress management, and emotional well-being in promoting health and vitality.

Key Principles of Dr. Barbara's Holistic Approach to Mucus Cleanse

Dr. Barbara's holistic approach to mucus cleanse is guided by several key principles:

1. **Nutritional Support**: A foundational aspect of mucus cleanse involves optimizing nutrition to support the body's natural detoxification processes. This includes consuming a diet rich in whole, nutrient-dense foods such as fruits, vegetables, lean proteins, healthy fats, and fiber. Avoidance of processed foods, refined sugars, and inflammatory ingredients is also emphasized to reduce mucus production and support overall health.

2. **Hydration**: Adequate hydration is essential for maintaining optimal mucus consistency and promoting its clearance from the body. Dr. Barbara recommends drinking plenty of water throughout the day to keep mucous membranes moist and facilitate the removal of excess mucus. Herbal teas, broths, and hydrating foods such as fruits and vegetables can also contribute to hydration and support mucus cleanse.

3. **Detoxification**: Supporting the body's natural detoxification pathways is a cornerstone of Dr. Barbara's holistic approach. This involves reducing exposure to environmental toxins and supporting liver, kidney, and lymphatic function through dietary and lifestyle interventions. Incorporating detoxifying foods and herbs, such as dandelion root, milk thistle, and cilantro, can aid in the elimination of toxins and promote mucus cleanse.

4. **Stress Management**: Chronic stress can impair immune function and exacerbate mucus-related symptoms. Dr. Barbara emphasizes the importance of stress management techniques such as mindfulness, meditation, deep breathing, and relaxation exercises to promote relaxation and reduce stress-related mucus production.

5. **Gut Health**: The health of the gastrointestinal tract plays a significant role in mucus production and overall well-being. Dr. Barbara's approach includes supporting gut health through probiotics, prebiotics, fermented foods, and digestive enzymes to optimize digestion, absorption, and elimination. Addressing gut imbalances such as dysbiosis, leaky gut, and food sensitivities can help reduce mucus production and promote healing.

6. **Herbal Medicine**: Herbal remedies are often used in conjunction with dietary and lifestyle interventions to support mucus cleanse and respiratory health. Dr. Barbara recommends specific herbs with expectorant, decongestant, and immune-enhancing properties, such as licorice root, ginger, turmeric, eucalyptus, and elderberry. These herbs can help loosen and expel mucus, soothe inflamed mucous membranes, and support immune function.

Benefits of Dr. Barbara's Holistic Approach to Mucus Cleanse

Adopting Dr. Barbara's holistic approach to mucus cleanse offers numerous benefits for overall health and well-being:

1. **Comprehensive Healing**: By addressing the root causes of mucus imbalance and supporting the body's innate healing mechanisms, holistic mucus cleanse promotes comprehensive healing on physical, mental, emotional, and spiritual levels.

2. **Individualized Care**: Dr. Barbara's approach recognizes that each person is unique, and there is no one-size-fits-all solution to mucus-related issues. By taking into account individual differences in genetics, physiology, lifestyle, and environment, holistic mucus cleanse can be tailored to meet the specific needs of each individual.

3. **Long-term Sustainability**: Unlike quick-fix approaches that focus on symptom relief without addressing underlying imbalances, holistic mucus cleanse promotes long-term sustainability by cultivating healthy habits and lifestyle practices that support ongoing health and vitality.

4. **Reduced Dependence on Medications**: By addressing root causes and promoting natural healing, holistic mucus cleanse may reduce the need for pharmaceutical interventions and

their associated side effects. Many individuals find that they can manage mucus-related symptoms more effectively through holistic approaches, thereby reducing reliance on medications.

5. **Improved Quality of Life**: By alleviating mucus-related symptoms such as congestion, coughing, sinusitis, and digestive issues, holistic mucus cleanse can significantly improve quality of life and overall well-being. Many individuals experience increased energy, vitality, and resilience as a result of adopting a holistic approach to mucus cleanse.

In conclusion, Dr. Barbara's holistic approach to mucus cleanse offers a comprehensive and effective way to address imbalances in the body that contribute to excessive mucus production. By integrating principles of nutrition, hydration, detoxification, stress management, gut health, and herbal medicine, this approach promotes healing on physical, mental, emotional, and spiritual levels. By addressing root causes and supporting the body's innate healing mechanisms, holistic mucus cleanse offers numerous benefits for overall health and well-being, including comprehensive healing, individualized care, long-term sustainability, reduced dependence on medications, and improved quality of life.

CHAPTER TWO

Understanding Mucus: Its Role in Health and Disease According to Dr. Barbara

Mucus, often overlooked in its significance, plays a pivotal role in maintaining health and preventing disease. Dr. Barbara, a renowned holistic health practitioner, emphasizes the importance of understanding mucus and its impact on the body's overall well-being. In this detailed exploration, we'll delve into the multifaceted role of mucus in health and disease, as elucidated by Dr. Barbara's perspective.

The Physiology of Mucus

Mucus is a viscous, gel-like substance produced by specialized cells in various mucous membranes throughout the body, including the respiratory, digestive, and reproductive tracts. It primarily consists of water, glycoproteins, lipids, and electrolytes, forming a protective barrier against pathogens, allergens, and irritants.

In the respiratory tract, mucus serves as a critical defense mechanism, trapping foreign particles and microbes and facilitating their removal via coughing, sneezing, or swallowing. In the digestive tract, mucus lubricates and protects the mucosal lining, aiding in the digestion and absorption of nutrients while preventing damage from digestive enzymes and acidic contents.

The Role of Mucus in Health

Mucus plays several essential roles in maintaining health and homeostasis:

1. **Protection**: Mucus acts as a physical barrier against pathogens, toxins, and mechanical damage, preventing infections and maintaining the integrity of mucous membranes.

2. **Moisturization**: Mucus lubricates and moisturizes various surfaces, including the respiratory and digestive tracts, preventing dryness and irritation.

3. **Immune Function**: Mucus contains immunoglobulins, enzymes, and antimicrobial peptides that help neutralize pathogens and modulate immune responses, contributing to overall immune function.

4. **Nutrient Absorption**: In the digestive tract, mucus facilitates the absorption of nutrients by protecting the mucosal lining and providing a conducive environment for enzymatic activity.

Imbalances in Mucus Production: Health Implications

While mucus is essential for maintaining health, imbalances in its production or composition can lead to various health issues:

1. **Excessive Mucus Production**: Overproduction of mucus, often triggered by factors such as infections, allergies, pollutants, or irritants, can lead to congestion, coughing, sinusitis, and respiratory discomfort.

2. **Thickened or Sticky Mucus**: Changes in the composition of mucus, such as increased viscosity or altered consistency, can impair its clearance from the body, leading to congestion, mucus plugs, and respiratory infections.

3. **Impaired Mucus Clearance**: Dysfunction of the mucociliary escalator, a mechanism responsible for moving mucus and trapped particles out of the respiratory tract, can impair mucus clearance and predispose individuals to respiratory infections and lung diseases.

4. **Inflammatory Conditions**: Chronic inflammation of mucous membranes, as seen in conditions like asthma, chronic bronchitis, and inflammatory bowel disease, can lead to increased mucus production, mucosal damage, and tissue remodeling.

Dr. Barbara's Perspective on Mucus-Related Health Issues

Dr. Barbara adopts a holistic approach to understanding and addressing mucus-related health issues, emphasizing the interconnectedness of body systems and the importance of addressing underlying imbalances. According to Dr. Barbara:

1. **Root Causes**: Rather than merely treating symptoms, it is essential to identify and address the root causes of mucus imbalances, which may include dietary factors, environmental toxins, stress, immune dysfunction, and microbial imbalances.

2. **Diet and Nutrition**: Nutrition plays a crucial role in mucus production and composition. Dr. Barbara advocates for a diet rich in whole, nutrient-dense foods, emphasizing fruits, vegetables, lean proteins, healthy fats, and hydration to support optimal mucus production and clearance.

3. **Detoxification**: Supporting the body's natural detoxification pathways, particularly those involving the liver, kidneys, and lymphatic system, can help reduce toxic burden and promote healthy mucus production and elimination.

4. **Stress Management**: Chronic stress can exacerbate mucus-related symptoms by dysregulating immune function and inflammatory responses. Stress management techniques such as mindfulness, meditation, and relaxation exercises are integral to Dr. Barbara's approach.

5. **Gut Health**: The health of the gastrointestinal tract influences mucus production and immune function. Dr.

Barbara emphasizes the importance of gut health, including probiotics, prebiotics, fiber, and digestive enzymes, in supporting mucus balance and overall well-being.

6. **Herbal Remedies**: Herbal medicine offers natural remedies to support mucus balance and respiratory health. Dr. Barbara recommends specific herbs with expectorant, anti-inflammatory, and immune-modulating properties, such as licorice root, ginger, turmeric, and marshmallow root.

Conclusion

In conclusion, mucus plays a vital role in maintaining health and preventing disease by protecting mucous membranes, facilitating immune function, and supporting nutrient absorption. Imbalances in mucus production or composition can lead to various health issues, including respiratory congestion, infections, and inflammatory conditions. Dr. Barbara's holistic approach to understanding and addressing mucus-related health issues emphasizes identifying and addressing underlying imbalances through diet, nutrition, detoxification, stress management, gut health, and herbal remedies. By adopting a comprehensive approach that addresses root causes and supports the body's innate healing mechanisms, individuals can promote optimal mucus balance and overall well-being.

CHAPTER THREE

The Science Behind Herbal Mucus Cleansing: How Herbs Aid Detoxification

Herbal mucus cleansing has been utilized for centuries as a natural approach to supporting the body's detoxification processes and promoting overall health and well-being. In this exploration, we'll delve into the scientific basis behind herbal mucus cleansing, examining how specific herbs aid in detoxification and mucus elimination according to modern research and traditional wisdom.

1. Herbal Expectorants and Decongestants

Many herbs possess expectorant and decongestant properties, making them valuable allies in promoting mucus clearance from the respiratory tract. These herbs work by:

- **Increasing Mucous Secretion**: Certain herbs stimulate the production of mucus in the respiratory tract, which can help thin and loosen existing mucus, making it easier to expel. This mechanism is particularly beneficial for individuals with thick or sticky mucus that is difficult to clear.

- **Enhancing Ciliary Action**: Cilia are tiny hair-like structures that line the respiratory tract and play a crucial role in moving mucus and trapped particles out of the airways.

Some herbs can enhance ciliary action, improving the efficiency of mucus clearance and reducing congestion.

- **Relaxing Bronchial Muscles**: Herbs with bronchodilator properties help relax the muscles surrounding the airways, facilitating easier breathing and mucus expulsion. This can be especially beneficial for individuals with asthma or bronchial spasms.

Common herbal expectorants and decongestants include:

- **Licorice Root (Glycyrrhiza glabra)**: Licorice root contains glycyrrhizin, a compound with expectorant properties that can help loosen and expel mucus from the respiratory tract. It also exhibits anti-inflammatory effects, which can help reduce airway inflammation and congestion.

- **Ginger (Zingiber officinale)**: Ginger is well-known for its ability to soothe digestive discomfort, but it also possesses expectorant and decongestant properties. Gingerols and shogaols, the active compounds in ginger, have been shown to stimulate mucus secretion and enhance ciliary activity, promoting mucus clearance.

- **Eucalyptus (Eucalyptus globulus)**: Eucalyptus contains cineole, a potent compound that acts as a mucolytic agent, helping to break down mucus and improve respiratory function. Inhalation of eucalyptus oil vapor has been shown to reduce nasal congestion and promote bronchial dilation.

- **Peppermint (Mentha piperita)**: Peppermint contains menthol, which has both decongestant and bronchodilator effects. Inhaling peppermint vapor or consuming peppermint tea can help alleviate nasal congestion and promote clearer breathing.

2. Anti-inflammatory and Antioxidant Effects

Chronic inflammation and oxidative stress play significant roles in mucus-related health issues, including respiratory congestion, sinusitis, and inflammatory bowel disease. Certain herbs exhibit potent anti-inflammatory and antioxidant effects, which can help reduce inflammation, protect mucous membranes, and support mucus balance.

- **Turmeric (Curcuma longa)**: Curcumin, the active compound in turmeric, is a potent anti-inflammatory and antioxidant agent. It modulates inflammatory pathways, inhibits the production of pro-inflammatory cytokines, and scavenges free radicals, thereby reducing mucosal inflammation and oxidative damage.

- **Marshmallow Root (Althaea officinalis)**: Marshmallow root contains mucilage, a gel-like substance that coats and soothes inflamed mucous membranes. It forms a protective barrier against irritants and promotes tissue repair, making it beneficial for conditions such as gastritis, esophagitis, and bronchitis.

- **Boswellia (Boswellia serrata)**: Boswellia contains boswellic acids, which possess anti-inflammatory and analgesic properties. It inhibits the production of inflammatory mediators such as leukotrienes and prostaglandins, reducing inflammation and promoting tissue healing in conditions such as asthma and inflammatory bowel disease.

3. Immunomodulatory Effects

A balanced immune response is essential for maintaining mucus balance and preventing excessive mucus production or inflammation. Certain herbs have immunomodulatory effects, helping to regulate immune function and promote a healthy inflammatory response.

- **Elderberry (Sambucus nigra)**: Elderberry is rich in flavonoids and anthocyanins, which have been shown to modulate immune function and inhibit viral replication. It supports the body's natural defenses against respiratory infections and may help reduce mucus production associated with colds and flu.

- **Astragalus (Astragalus membranaceus)**: Astragalus contains polysaccharides and saponins that enhance immune function and stimulate the production of interferons and other antiviral compounds. It strengthens respiratory immunity and may help reduce mucus-related symptoms in individuals prone to recurrent infections.

Conclusion

Herbal mucus cleansing is supported by scientific evidence demonstrating the efficacy of specific herbs in promoting mucus clearance, reducing inflammation, and supporting immune function. By incorporating herbal expectorants, decongestants, anti-inflammatory agents, antioxidants, and immunomodulators into a holistic approach to mucus cleanse, individuals can support their body's natural detoxification processes and promote respiratory health. However, it's essential to consult with a qualified healthcare practitioner before using herbal remedies, especially if you have underlying health conditions or are taking medications.

CHAPTER FOUR

Preparing for the Cleanse: Steps to Take Before Starting Dr. Barbara's 7-Day Program

Embarking on Dr. Barbara's 7-day cleanse program can be a transformative journey towards revitalizing your health and well-being. However, proper preparation is essential to ensure a smooth and successful experience. In this guide, we'll outline the steps you should take before starting Dr. Barbara's cleanse program to maximize its effectiveness and minimize any potential discomfort.

1. Consultation with a Healthcare Professional

Before beginning any new health regimen, it's crucial to consult with a qualified healthcare professional, especially if you have underlying health conditions or are taking medications. Your healthcare provider can provide personalized guidance based on your individual health status and help you determine if Dr. Barbara's cleanse program is suitable for you.

2. Set Clear Intentions and Goals

Take some time to reflect on your reasons for embarking on Dr. Barbara's cleanse program and set clear intentions and goals for what you hope to achieve. Whether you're seeking to improve digestion, boost energy levels, or kickstart healthier habits, having a clear vision of your objectives will help you stay motivated and focused throughout the cleanse.

3. Educate Yourself on the Cleanse Protocol

Familiarize yourself with the details of Dr. Barbara's 7-day cleanse program, including the recommended dietary guidelines, herbal supplements, and lifestyle practices involved. Understanding the rationale behind each component of the cleanse will empower you to make informed choices and adhere to the protocol more effectively.

4. Prepare Your Environment

Create a supportive environment conducive to cleansing by removing temptations and distractions that may derail your progress. Stock your kitchen with nutrient-dense whole foods, herbal supplements, and cleansing teas recommended by Dr. Barbara. Clear your schedule as much as possible to minimize stress and prioritize self-care during the cleanse week.

5. Gradually Transition to a Cleanse-Friendly Diet

Ease your body into the cleanse process by gradually transitioning to a cleanse-friendly diet in the days leading up to the start of the program. Focus on consuming whole, plant-based foods such as fruits, vegetables, whole grains, legumes, nuts, and seeds while minimizing processed foods, refined sugars, caffeine, alcohol, and animal products. This gradual approach will help minimize detox symptoms and prepare your body for the more restrictive phase of the cleanse.

6. Hydrate and Support Elimination Pathways

Hydration is essential for supporting the body's natural detoxification processes, so be sure to drink plenty of water throughout the day. Additionally, incorporate hydrating foods such as cucumbers, watermelon, celery, and citrus fruits into your diet to promote hydration and support the elimination of toxins.

7. Practice Mindfulness and Stress Management

Cleansing is not just about detoxifying the body; it's also an opportunity to nourish your mind and spirit. Incorporate mindfulness practices such as meditation, deep breathing, yoga, or journaling into your daily routine to reduce stress, promote relaxation, and cultivate a positive mindset. Prioritizing self-care and stress management will enhance the overall effectiveness of Dr. Barbara's cleanse program.

8. Gather Supplies and Resources

Ensure that you have all the necessary supplies and resources on hand before starting Dr. Barbara's cleanse program. This may include herbal supplements, cleansing teas, organic produce, kitchen essentials for meal preparation, and any supportive materials or resources provided as part of the cleanse program.

9. Enlist Support and Accountability

Embarking on a cleanse program can be challenging, especially if you're making significant dietary and lifestyle changes. Enlist the support of friends, family members, or a cleanse buddy who can offer encouragement, accountability, and companionship throughout the cleanse journey. Having a support system in place will increase your likelihood of success and make the experience more enjoyable.

By following these preparatory steps, you'll set yourself up for a successful and transformative experience with Dr. Barbara's 7-day cleanse program. Remember to approach the cleanse with an open mind, listen to your body's signals, and honor your unique needs throughout the process.

CHAPTER FIVE

Day 1: Initiating the Cleanse with Herbal Remedies to Clear Mucus Buildup

Congratulations on embarking on Dr. Barbara's cleanse program! Day 1 marks the beginning of your journey towards detoxification and revitalization. Today, we'll focus on initiating the cleanse with herbal remedies specifically designed to clear mucus buildup from the body. These herbal remedies will support your body's natural detoxification processes and help kickstart the cleansing process.

1. Start Your Day with Warm Lemon Water

Upon waking up, begin your day with a glass of warm lemon water. Lemon water helps alkalize the body, supports liver function, and stimulates digestion, making it an excellent choice to kickstart your cleanse. Squeeze the juice of half a lemon into a glass of warm water and drink it on an empty stomach before consuming any other foods or beverages.

2. Herbal Expectorant Tea Blend

Throughout the day, sip on an herbal expectorant tea blend to help loosen and expel mucus from the respiratory tract. Prepare a tea using a combination of herbs known for their expectorant properties, such as:

- Licorice root: Soothes irritated mucous membranes and supports respiratory health.

- Ginger: Has expectorant and anti-inflammatory properties, helping to clear congestion.

- Marshmallow root: Contains mucilage, which coats and soothes inflamed tissues, promoting mucus clearance.

- Eucalyptus: Acts as a decongestant and helps open up the airways for easier breathing.

Steep the herbs in hot water for 5-10 minutes, then strain and enjoy the tea throughout the day. You can sweeten it with a little raw honey if desired.

3. Incorporate Mucus-Clearing Foods into Your Meals

Focus on consuming mucus-clearing foods as part of your meals today. These include:

- Fruits: Particularly citrus fruits like oranges, grapefruits, and lemons, which are high in vitamin C and help thin mucus.

- Vegetables: Dark leafy greens, cruciferous vegetables (broccoli, cabbage, kale), and peppers are rich in antioxidants and support detoxification.

- Garlic and onions: These aromatic vegetables have antimicrobial properties and can help clear mucus from the respiratory tract.

- Spices: Turmeric, cayenne pepper, and black pepper have anti-inflammatory properties and may help reduce mucus production.

Incorporate these foods into your meals in creative ways, such as adding citrus segments to salads, including garlic and onions in stir-fries, or seasoning dishes with turmeric and cayenne pepper.

4. Herbal Respiratory Steam Inhalation

In the evening, treat yourself to a herbal respiratory steam inhalation to further clear congestion and promote mucus elimination. Boil a pot of water and add a few drops of essential oils or dried herbs with decongestant properties, such as eucalyptus, peppermint, or thyme. Cover your head with a towel and lean over the pot, inhaling the steam deeply for 5-10 minutes. Be careful to avoid getting too close to the hot water to prevent burns.

5. Hydrate and Rest

Throughout the day, prioritize hydration by drinking plenty of water, herbal teas, and hydrating fluids. Adequate hydration supports the body's detoxification processes and helps thin mucus for easier elimination. Additionally, prioritize rest and relaxation to support your body's healing and rejuvenation during the cleanse.

By incorporating these herbal remedies and mucus-clearing practices into your Day 1 routine, you'll lay a solid foundation for clearing mucus buildup from your body and jumpstarting your cleanse journey with Dr. Barbara. Stay committed to the process, listen to your body's signals, and trust in the healing power of nature as you embark on this transformative experience.

CHAPTER SIX

Days 2-5: Deepening the Cleanse with Specific Herbs and Nutrients

As you progress through Dr. Barbara's cleanse program, days 2 to 5 are pivotal for deepening the detoxification process and supporting your body's natural healing mechanisms. During this phase, we'll focus on incorporating specific herbs and nutrients known for their detoxifying and mucus-clearing properties to further enhance the cleanse. Here's a comprehensive guide to help you navigate days 2 to 5 of the cleanse:

1. Continue with Herbal Expectorant Tea Blend

Maintain your daily intake of the herbal expectorant tea blend introduced on Day 1. Sip on this tea throughout the day to continue supporting mucus clearance from the respiratory tract. Consistency is key to maximizing the benefits of these herbal remedies.

2. Introduce Detoxifying Herbs and Nutrients

In addition to the herbal expectorant tea blend, incorporate detoxifying herbs and nutrients into your daily routine to further support the cleanse process. Consider adding the following supplements or foods rich in detoxifying compounds:

- **Milk Thistle**: This herb supports liver health and detoxification by promoting the production of glutathione, a powerful antioxidant enzyme. Take milk thistle supplements or include it in your diet through herbal teas or tinctures.

- **Dandelion Root**: Dandelion root stimulates liver function and enhances bile production, facilitating the elimination of toxins from the body. Enjoy dandelion root tea or incorporate fresh dandelion greens into your salads or smoothies.

- **N-acetylcysteine (NAC)**: NAC is a precursor to glutathione, a key antioxidant involved in detoxification. Consider taking NAC supplements to support glutathione production and enhance detoxification pathways.

- **Cruciferous Vegetables**: Broccoli, cauliflower, Brussels sprouts, and cabbage contain compounds called glucosinolates, which support liver detoxification processes. Incorporate these vegetables into your meals regularly.

- **Chlorella and Spirulina**: These nutrient-dense algae are rich in chlorophyll and antioxidants, supporting detoxification and cellular health. Add chlorella or spirulina powder to smoothies or take them as supplements.

3. Emphasize Whole, Plant-Based Foods

During days 2 to 5 of the cleanse, prioritize whole, plant-based foods that support detoxification and mucus clearance. Incorporate a variety of fruits, vegetables, legumes, nuts, seeds, and whole grains into your meals to provide essential nutrients and fiber for optimal digestion and elimination.

4. Hydration and Electrolyte Balance

Continue to prioritize hydration by drinking plenty of water, herbal teas, and electrolyte-rich fluids such as coconut water. Proper hydration is essential for supporting detoxification pathways and maintaining electrolyte balance in the body.

5. Gentle Movement and Exercise

Engage in gentle movement and exercise to support circulation, lymphatic drainage, and overall well-being during the cleanse. Activities such as walking, yoga, stretching, and tai chi can promote relaxation and facilitate the elimination of toxins from the body.

6. Mindful Eating and Stress Management

Practice mindful eating and stress management techniques to support digestion, reduce inflammation, and promote overall relaxation. Take time to chew your food thoroughly, savoring each bite, and minimize distractions during meals. Incorporate stress-reducing practices such as meditation, deep breathing, and journaling to promote emotional balance and enhance the cleanse experience.

7. Monitor Your Progress and Adjust as Needed

Pay attention to how your body responds to the cleanse and make adjustments as needed based on your individual experience. If you experience any adverse reactions or discomfort, consult with a healthcare professional for guidance. Listen to your body's signals and honor its needs throughout the cleanse journey.

By deepening the cleanse with specific herbs and nutrients during days 2 to 5, you'll support your body's detoxification processes and further enhance mucus clearance. Stay committed to the program, prioritize self-care, and trust in the healing power of nature as you continue on your cleanse journey with Dr. Barbara.

CHAPTER SEVEN

Day 6: Revitalizing the Body as the Cleanse Progresses

As you approach the final stretch of Dr. Barbara's cleanse program, Day 6 presents an opportunity to revitalize your body and prepare for the transition back to regular eating habits. Today, we'll focus on nourishing the body with revitalizing foods, incorporating gentle movement and self-care practices, and reflecting on the progress you've made throughout the cleanse. Here's how to make the most of Day 6:

1. Nutrient-Rich, Whole Foods

Transition from the more restrictive phase of the cleanse to incorporating a wider variety of nutrient-rich, whole foods into your meals. Focus on incorporating fresh fruits, vegetables, leafy greens, whole grains, legumes, nuts, seeds, and lean proteins to provide essential nutrients and support overall vitality.

2. Incorporate Superfoods and Antioxidants

Boost your intake of superfoods and antioxidants to further support cellular health and detoxification. Consider adding foods such as berries, dark leafy greens, turmeric, ginger, chia seeds, flaxseeds, and walnuts to your meals to provide a rich source of vitamins, minerals, and phytonutrients.

3. Herbal Tonics and Elixirs

Indulge in herbal tonics and elixirs to nourish and rejuvenate your body from within. Prepare a revitalizing tonic using adaptogenic herbs such as ashwagandha, rhodiola, holy basil, and maca to support adrenal health, balance stress hormones, and promote energy and vitality.

4. Gentle Movement and Exercise

Engage in gentle movement and exercise to promote circulation, flexibility, and overall well-being. Consider activities such as yoga, qigong, walking in nature, or gentle stretching to invigorate your body and reduce stress. Listen to your body's cues and choose activities that feel nurturing and supportive.

5. Self-Care and Relaxation

Prioritize self-care and relaxation to rejuvenate your mind, body, and spirit. Take time to indulge in activities that bring you joy and nourishment, whether it's reading a book, taking a bath, practicing meditation, or spending time in nature. Cultivate an atmosphere of calm and serenity to support your body's healing and renewal.

6. Reflect on Your Cleanse Journey

Take a moment to reflect on the progress you've made throughout the cleanse journey. Celebrate your achievements, no matter how small, and acknowledge the dedication and commitment you've shown to your health and well-being. Use this time for introspection and gratitude as you prepare to transition back to your regular routine.

7. Stay Hydrated and Rested

Continue to prioritize hydration by drinking plenty of water, herbal teas, and hydrating fluids throughout the day. Adequate hydration supports detoxification and revitalization, helping to flush out toxins and replenish essential fluids in the body. Additionally, prioritize rest and relaxation to allow your body to recharge and rejuvenate as you near the end of the cleanse.

8. Prepare for the Transition

Start preparing for the transition back to regular eating habits by gradually reintroducing foods that were restricted during the cleanse. Begin with easily digestible foods such as steamed vegetables, soups, and lean proteins, and slowly reintroduce other foods while paying attention to how your body responds.

By revitalizing the body on Day 6 of Dr. Barbara's cleanse program, you'll nourish your body, mind, and spirit as you prepare for the final day of the cleanse and beyond. Stay present, embrace the journey, and continue to prioritize your health and well-being as you approach the culmination of this transformative experience.

CHAPTER EIGHT

Day 7: Completing the Cleanse and Transitioning Back to Regular Eating

Congratulations on reaching Day 7 of Dr. Barbara's cleanse program! Today marks the culmination of your journey towards detoxification, rejuvenation, and renewed vitality. As you complete the cleanse, it's essential to approach this final day with mindfulness and intentionality, ensuring a smooth transition back to regular eating habits. Here's how to navigate Day 7 and transition back to a balanced, nourishing diet:

1. Reflect on Your Cleanse Experience

Take some time to reflect on your cleanse experience and the progress you've made throughout the past week. Acknowledge any insights, challenges, or breakthroughs you've experienced and celebrate your commitment to prioritizing your health and well-being. Use this reflection as an opportunity for growth and self-awareness as you move forward.

2. Hydrate and Flush Toxins

Continue to prioritize hydration by drinking plenty of water, herbal teas, and hydrating fluids throughout the day. Hydration supports the body's detoxification processes, helping to flush out toxins and promote overall vitality. Aim to drink at least eight glasses of water or more, depending on your individual needs.

3. Incorporate Whole, Nutrient-Dense Foods

As you transition back to regular eating habits, focus on incorporating whole, nutrient-dense foods into your meals. Emphasize fruits, vegetables, leafy greens, whole grains, legumes, nuts, seeds, and lean proteins to provide essential nutrients and support overall health and vitality. Choose foods that nourish and energize your body, avoiding processed and refined foods.

4. Gradually Reintroduce Foods

Begin by reintroducing foods that were restricted during the cleanse gradually. Start with easily digestible foods such as steamed vegetables, soups, salads, and whole grains, and gradually reintroduce other foods while paying attention to how your body responds. Notice any sensitivities or reactions and adjust your diet accordingly.

5. Practice Mindful Eating

Cultivate mindfulness around your eating habits by paying attention to hunger cues, eating slowly, and savoring each bite. Tune in to your body's signals of hunger and satiety, and honor its needs with nourishing, balanced meals. Avoid distractions such as screens or multitasking during meals to fully appreciate and enjoy your food.

6. Support Digestion

Support your digestive system as you transition back to regular eating habits by incorporating foods and practices that promote optimal digestion. Consider including fermented foods such as yogurt, kefir, sauerkraut, and kombucha to support gut health and aid digestion. Additionally, enjoy herbal teas such as ginger, peppermint, or fennel after meals to soothe the digestive tract.

7. Continue Self-Care Practices

Maintain self-care practices that support your overall well-being, including stress management techniques, relaxation exercises, and regular movement or exercise. Prioritize activities that nourish your mind, body, and spirit, and create a supportive environment conducive to health and vitality.

8. Set Intentions for Continued Health

As you complete the cleanse and transition back to regular eating habits, set intentions for continued health and well-being moving forward. Commit to making conscious choices that support your health, such as nourishing your body with wholesome foods, staying hydrated, managing stress effectively, and prioritizing self-care.

By completing Dr. Barbara's cleanse program with mindfulness and intentionality, you'll emerge feeling refreshed, rejuvenated, and empowered to continue prioritizing your health and well-being in the days and weeks ahead. Embrace this opportunity for growth and transformation, and trust in your body's innate ability to thrive.

CHAPTER NINE

Navigating Detox Symptoms: Tips for Overcoming Challenges During the Cleanse

Embarking on a cleanse journey can be a transformative experience, but it's not uncommon to encounter detox symptoms along the way. These symptoms may include fatigue, headaches, digestive disturbances, mood swings, and skin breakouts as the body releases accumulated toxins and undergoes purification. While these symptoms can be challenging, they are often temporary and signify the body's natural healing and detoxification process. Here are some tips to help you navigate detox symptoms and overcome challenges during the cleanse:

1. Stay Hydrated

Proper hydration is essential for supporting detoxification and minimizing detox symptoms. Drink plenty of water, herbal teas, and electrolyte-rich fluids throughout the day to help flush out toxins and replenish essential fluids in the body. Aim to drink at least eight glasses of water per day, or more if you're experiencing increased sweating or detoxification.

2. Rest and Relaxation

Give your body the rest and relaxation it needs to support the cleansing process. Prioritize sleep and aim for at least 7-8 hours of quality sleep each night to promote healing and rejuvenation.

Incorporate relaxation techniques such as meditation, deep breathing exercises, or gentle stretching to reduce stress and promote overall well-being.

3. Supportive Nutrition

Focus on nourishing your body with nutrient-dense, whole foods that support detoxification and provide essential nutrients. Incorporate plenty of fruits, vegetables, leafy greens, whole grains, legumes, nuts, seeds, and lean proteins into your meals to provide essential vitamins, minerals, and antioxidants. Avoid processed foods, refined sugars, caffeine, alcohol, and inflammatory foods that may exacerbate detox symptoms.

4. Herbal Support

Utilize herbal remedies to support your body's natural detoxification processes and alleviate detox symptoms. Consider incorporating herbs such as dandelion root, milk thistle, burdock root, ginger, turmeric, and peppermint into your daily routine to support liver function, promote digestion, and reduce inflammation. Herbal teas, tinctures, or supplements can be beneficial for providing targeted support during the cleanse.

5. Gentle Exercise

Engage in gentle exercise and movement to promote circulation, lymphatic drainage, and overall well-being. Activities such as walking, yoga, tai chi, or swimming can help stimulate the lymphatic system, support detoxification, and reduce stress. Listen to your body and choose activities that feel nourishing and supportive during the cleanse.

6. Manage Stress

Stress can exacerbate detox symptoms and hinder the body's natural healing processes. Practice stress management techniques such as meditation, deep breathing exercises, mindfulness, or spending time in nature to reduce stress and promote relaxation. Prioritize self-care activities that bring you joy and support your emotional well-being throughout the cleanse.

7. Listen to Your Body

Pay attention to your body's signals and adjust your cleanse protocol as needed based on how you're feeling. If you're experiencing severe or prolonged detox symptoms, consider slowing down the cleanse process, reducing the intensity of detoxifying practices, or seeking guidance from a qualified healthcare professional. Honor your body's needs and trust its innate wisdom as you navigate the cleansing journey.

8. Seek Support

Don't hesitate to seek support from friends, family members, or a healthcare practitioner if you're feeling overwhelmed or uncertain during the cleanse. Having a supportive community can provide encouragement, accountability, and guidance as you navigate detox symptoms and overcome challenges along the way. Reach out for assistance when needed and remember that you're not alone on this journey.

By implementing these tips, you can effectively navigate detox symptoms and overcome challenges during the cleanse, ultimately supporting your body's natural healing and purification process. Embrace the journey with patience, compassion, and resilience, knowing that each step brings you closer to renewed vitality and well-being.

CHAPTER TEN

Integrating Herbal Mucus Cleansing into Your Lifestyle for Ongoing Health and Wellness

Herbal mucus cleansing offers numerous benefits for overall health and wellness, and integrating these practices into your lifestyle can support ongoing detoxification, respiratory health, and vitality. By incorporating herbal remedies, dietary modifications, and lifestyle practices into your daily routine, you can maintain a healthy balance of mucus and promote optimal well-being. Here's how to integrate herbal mucus cleansing into your lifestyle for ongoing health and wellness:

1. Establish a Daily Herbal Routine

Incorporate herbal remedies known for their mucus-clearing properties into your daily routine to support respiratory health and detoxification. Brew herbal teas containing expectorant herbs such as licorice root, ginger, eucalyptus, and peppermint and enjoy them throughout the day. Additionally, consider taking herbal supplements or tinctures formulated to support respiratory health and mucus clearance on a regular basis.

2. Eat a Mucus-Balancing Diet

Adopt a mucus-balancing diet rich in whole, plant-based foods that support detoxification and respiratory health. Emphasize fruits, vegetables, leafy greens, whole grains, legumes, nuts, seeds, and lean proteins in your meals to provide essential nutrients and promote mucus balance. Minimize consumption of processed foods, refined sugars, dairy products, and inflammatory foods that may contribute to mucus buildup and inflammation.

3. Stay Hydrated

Maintain adequate hydration by drinking plenty of water, herbal teas, and hydrating fluids throughout the day. Proper hydration supports detoxification, helps thin mucus for easier elimination, and promotes overall health and vitality. Aim to drink at least eight glasses of water per day, or more if you're physically active or experiencing increased mucus production.

4. Practice Respiratory Health Maintenance

Incorporate practices that support respiratory health and maintain clear airways on a regular basis. Practice deep breathing exercises, steam inhalation with essential oils, and nasal irrigation using a saline solution to promote mucus clearance and relieve congestion. Additionally, avoid exposure to environmental pollutants, allergens, and irritants that may exacerbate respiratory symptoms.

5. Engage in Regular Exercise

Engage in regular exercise and physical activity to support circulation, lymphatic drainage, and overall well-being. Choose activities that promote cardiovascular health, such as walking, jogging, swimming, or cycling, and incorporate strength training and flexibility exercises into your routine. Exercise helps stimulate the lymphatic system, support detoxification, and reduce stress, contributing to overall health and wellness.

6. Prioritize Stress Management

Manage stress effectively to support immune function, reduce inflammation, and promote overall wellness. Incorporate stress management techniques such as meditation, yoga, deep breathing exercises, or mindfulness practices into your daily routine. Additionally, prioritize self-care activities that bring you joy and relaxation, such as spending time in nature, practicing hobbies, or connecting with loved ones.

7. Listen to Your Body

Pay attention to your body's signals and adjust your lifestyle habits as needed to maintain optimal health and wellness. Honor your body's needs for rest, nourishment, movement, and relaxation, and prioritize self-care practices that support your overall well-being. Trust your intuition and listen to your body's wisdom as you navigate your wellness journey.

8. Seek Professional Guidance

Consult with a qualified healthcare practitioner or herbalist for personalized guidance and support in integrating herbal mucus cleansing into your lifestyle. They can provide recommendations tailored to your individual health needs, help you select appropriate herbs and supplements, and monitor your progress over time. Working with a healthcare professional ensures that you receive safe and effective guidance for ongoing health and wellness.

By integrating herbal mucus cleansing into your lifestyle, you can support ongoing detoxification, respiratory health, and vitality, ultimately promoting optimal well-being and longevity. Embrace these practices with consistency, patience, and mindfulness, knowing that each step contributes to your overall health and wellness journey.

THE END

www.ingramcontent.com/pod-product-compliance
Lightning Source LLC
Chambersburg PA
CBHW081604250726
48653CB00009B/3555